Part 1:
Talk To Your Doctor

It's either because of your body or your brain. The end. That simple. (drops mic)

(picks mic back up)

Preface #1

First, let me say that many sexual issues regarding libido and performance can be attributed to health, medical issues and the medication taken to address those issues. If you even SUSPECT that this might be the case with you, it is infinitely better to address this with your Primary Care Physician (PCP) than taking advice over the internet. No matter how knowledgeable someone may seem, or actually how knowledgeable they may be, and how helpful they are, it is no substitute for the one-on-one relationship with a medical professional who gets to know you and can build an overview of all your complete medical and health needs and concerns.

Seriously. Talk to your doctor.

I am one such a knowledgeable someone and I always try to be helpful with the information I publish It is well researched and well vetted, confirmed with professionals and other such knowledgeable people.

Still. Talk to your doctor if you have ANY suspicion that there is a medical issue that is effecting your sex life. Sexual performance is a VERY good marker for many seemingly unrelated health issues that might go undetected otherwise until they are more serious.

I am not WebMD and will not give you a list of those medical conditions, issues, situations, maladies, illnesses and sicknesses so you can draw conclusions based on very general possibilities. Don't ask.

I will, however, go out on a limb and state that diet and exercise are a major factor. If you are overweight, your sex life can be effected greatly. If you are under exercised, same. A little cardio goes a long way. Smaller portions of food at a time. WHAT you eat is less of an issue than many people claim, as long as you don't eat too much of it at a time. Drink plenty of plain ol' water every single day too. For optimum health, a person should drink a 1/2 ounce of water for every pound of body weight. That sounds like a lot. But, try it. It's not as hard to do as that sounds.

This is true of men AND women. ALL men and women.

And talk to your doctor. Your doctor should know that you eat too much, don't drink enough water and don't get enough exercise. Of course, the more often you're at the doctor's office, the more likely your doctor already knows. Jus' sayin'.

There are also certain drugs well known for killing libido and performance. Anything for anxiety and/or depression, as well as a list of conditions in a similar arena are notorious for their effect on people's sex life. It doesn't necessarily have to be a sexual death sentence though. Meds can often be adjusted. Talk to your doctor.

If your doctor can't help you, as some doctors are reluctant to do, find another doctor who will be more open minded to making adjustments. Sometimes, to keep you sane and functioning, there might be limits to what adjustments can be made. And, your insurance company might have a say-so in some of the choices available. Still, this all begins with a conversation with a doctor who is willing to consider possibilities and options other than what is automatic.

Did I mention exercise? You don't have to become a gym rat. But I cannot emphasize it enough that a little cardio goes a long way. Men AND women. Orgasm might take place in the brain, but SEX involves the body. Respiration and circulation combined with a little mobility. The better you can move and the better you can breathe, the better your sex life will be.

Now, I will also share a little about menopause and hysterectomies - not as a medical professional, but as someone with some experience with the two.

The medical community will generally tell you that menopause usually marks a drastic decline in libido and sexual function due to the decline in production of the hormones and the chemistry involved. They also state that women's libidos peak between 30 and 40 and after that, well, welcome to menopause. My own experience with a surprising number of women who have had one and/or been through the other does not entirely confirm the accepted beliefs.

When I was in grad school, I had a FWB named Brenda who had received a full hysterectomy after giving birth to her son when she was 19. At the time, she was 26. She told me that before her surgery, she was almost uncontrollably horny all the time. "Maddening" was the word she used. Difficulty focusing in school or at work. Crazy horny, all the time. After the surgery, nothing. Even with HRT, nothing.

"Are you telling me you're never really horny? Why do we have sex then?" I asked her.

She giggled. "I have sex with you because I LIKE you and LIKE having sex with you. Just because my body doesn't get horny like that anymore doesn't mean I don't like being with you."

I was confused. Still young and very much driven by physical horniness, I needed a better explanation.

"I still have the emotional and mental drives," she told me. "I still NEED to be loved and held and feel desired, And sex still feels great and I have plenty of orgasms. I just don't have the physical drive to go get laid very much anymore."

Because I have been with several other women who have had a full hysterectomy, all of those in their 40s and 50s, I'm wondering if Brenda was the exception to the rule. If maybe SHE (and other women like her) is the reason the medical community holds the opinion they do.

Yes, a full hysterectomy causes a complete change in the hormones that form a lot of sexuality in women. But, the other women I have been with claimed that there was little difference between HRT and their pre-surgery level of libido and performance. A few even said HRT restored their hormone levels to where they were when they were younger, and now, they are as horny as teenagers. Not braggin', just sayin', these women were all multi-orgasmic when we were together. There wasn't quite as much natural lubrication as a younger woman. But other than that, sex seemed pretty normal. Granted, this is a small anecdotal group to make a conclusion about. But, it's enough that it makes me wonder if the accepted medical conclusion is as accurate as is believed. (shrugs)

HRT includes a wide range of medications. If you have any question about being on the right one(s), talk to your doctor. If you rarely get aroused or have difficulty with reaching an orgasm, your HRT medication MIGHT be the cause. I wonder, in hindsight, if that was the situation with Brenda. She needed her meds adjusted and no one figured that out. The doctor is not a mindreader. If Brenda didn't know there was a problem, how would she know to ask? And, if all the other symptoms seem to be addressed satisfactorily, why would anyone think to ask? So, they both think everything is the way it's supposed to be even though it definitely isn't. Talk to your doctor.

Since my early 40s, most of the women around my age I have played with in some way, or the ones I have worked with in a therapeutic way, have stated some level of experience with menopause or peri-menopause. Some were on HRT. Others used herbal remedies. And still others, just rode it out without anything. In this group, there was SOME decline in horniness, arousal took a little more foreplay, but overall, they were still quite sexual.

It could be very situational, possibly. I know that a hysterectomy and/or menopause doesn't make a woman feel sexy. There's a HUGE adjustment, mentally and emotionally, to a new normal. That feeling might have had a greater effect than the perceived medical situation. Maybe it's still blamed on menopause, but it's possibly the emotions that create the symptoms, not the physiology. I wonder.

I will also state that there are many emotional and mental factors that play a role with women's libidos and performance. Sometimes, those factors can present as actual physical issues. I'm not saying anyone is crazy or unstable. I'm saying that as a woman ages, her emotional and mental needs to get aroused and perform sexually change, possibly without other signs. So, she might be thinking peri-menopause and see her doctor, go on HRT and it doesn't help. Turns out, reducing stress and needing a little more romance in her life is the cure. Not meds.

There is also something I call "functional depression" that seems quite common. There are several ways that is diagnosed and treated, WHEN it is diagnosed. On the outside, the patient doesn't APPEAR depressed by classic measures. On the inside though, there is definitely some melancholy afoot. It may not even be apparent to a professional in the first conversation.

You can start with a conversation with your doctor and he/she will refer you to someone. Or, just call a few therapists and set up an appointment. Finding the right therapist is a lot like dating. Some will not be right for you and you'll discover that in the first session. There is nothing wrong with shopping / dating around a little. Once you find the right therapist, trust your gut. You'll know. Talking to a therapist is NEVER a bad idea.

This is why that, when you talk to your doctor, you tell the doctor EVERYTHING. Make the doctor listen, because I know that at times they seem rushed to get to the next patient. In their defense, they are quicker to dismiss a patient when the patient doesn't start talking. "Everything's fine? Okay. Next!!"

Tell your doctor EVERYTHING. Did I say that? I mean EVERYTHING. Even the stuff that doesn't seem related. Even the stuff that doesn't seem like anything. Even minor things can be related to major things. The more information you can give the doctor, the better they will be at helping you figure it all out. EVERYTHING.

Part 2:
Conditioning & What's Up

Now, if you are fairly certain that your issue does NOT have a medical or health related cause (And seriously. You should not be making that determination without your PCP in the conversation), then that only leaves the brain. THAT is something I'm more qualified to talk about and would like to offer some of my helpyness.

THAT is the purpose of this series.

Preface #2

Let me start with the part of this that will piss off a few of you. For the purpose of this article, I need to clarify some terms.

If you were born in a female body and were raised, up to puberty, as a female, appearing female to the world at large, regardless of your own personal identity as non binary, non-conforming, gender fluid, male, or anything else, the world saw you as a female and that's how you were conditioned to see the world back.

If you were born in a male body and were raised, up to puberty, as a male, appearing male to the world at large, regardless of your own identity as non binary, non-conforming, gender fluid, female, or anything else, the world saw you as a male and that's how you were conditioned to see the world back.

Same thing with gay or straight. As a child, almost everyone fits into the traditional straight models - even if you "felt" that didn't fit you. And thus, the world automatically assumes that you are straight and treats you like you are straight and conditions you as a straight person. I mean, who would know? Right?

Yes, I understand that people are not so simple and that identity and attraction are FAR more complicated than the traditional binary system. However, the world in general does not see it that way. We're better than we have ever been. But still, the world at large doesn't dig very deep and doesn't bother to learn more about anyone who APPEARS to fit one of the two traditional sets. And the truth is, the world doesn't care much until you start acting "weird", which includes any kind of appearance or behavior that doesn't fit the two, non-open-minded, traditional sets. Most kids, before puberty, don't usually do a whole lot of stuff that would be classified as "weird" in this context.

Regardless of where things went later, most people, act and appear, and were treated by the world, as part of this very narrow two-set system. Even if your parents knew you didn't fit one of those sets, the world around you didn't know and so you were treated as one or the other. Period.

I only get into this because even if you are gay, trans, born into the wrong body, pansexual, asexual or fit into any set that I have missed, your worldly conditioning - regardless of parental influence - is HEAVILY steered towards these two sets. HEAVILY. Did I say that? And because your impressionable psyche was so heavily influenced by the world at large and firmly driven into the two boxes, I am going to focus this discussion on those two sets because regardless of who you are later, as a child, these two sets are almost exclusively what you were taught.

And what you were taught THEN, is what decides your fate NOW. Even though, as a sexually active adult, you are not even close to the standard you were handed as a child, that programming you received by the world at large is still a major part of how you do things. Those first few years, up to about 10, 11 or 12 or so, decided so much of how you think about sex, even though you (probably) weren't sexualized by then.

BTW. Stop. If you're going to send me an email telling me that YOU were very sexual at a younger age or that you knew you were gay at a younger age, or you want to tell me that your family knew and treated you respectfully by your true self, don't. Just don't. I already know that's true of some people. If you are one of those some people, that's fine. It still doesn't change how the world probably treated you. It still doesn't change your worldly conditioning by the majority of the world around you.

It is how the world conditioned you that makes it necessary for this article to focus on the narrow, two-set system. Almost everyone was conditioned based on this system. Almost. Everyone. Even you.

All that said, let's see if we can answer that original question. Okay?

So, we have cleared the medical threshold and accepted that almost everyone, for the first decade or so of their life, was raised in a very narrow male or female system. Good. Let me begin now. Let's start with a little neurology of how things are supposed to work. Shall we?

Men's brains and women's brains are slightly different. Well, they WORK slightly different. Literally. They work differently in very subtle ways that can have enormous results. Blame evolution for that. Men and women evolved to fulfill different roles in ensuring the survival of the tribe and it shows in the subtle differences in how our brains process information. There are quite a few reputable studies that have covered this. These differences don't always seem HUGE, even though they can have a HUGE impact on behavior and our perception of the world around us.

During sex, both brains act a lot alike in many ways. In both, the lateral orbitofrontal cortex, which controls reason and behavior, shuts down during orgasm. So, to describe an orgasm as being "out of control", it's very accurate. But, the periaqueductal gray in women is far more active. The PAG has enkephalin-producing cells that suppress pain. At the same time, the area of the cortex that is associated with pain is also quite active. The relationship between these two being active in such a way is unclear.

My personal opinion is that the cortex makes a woman more sensitive to pain, while the PAG reduces that pain, leaving her body way more sensitive in general to a wide range of other sensations. My personal observations would confirm that, as well as many, many, many testimonials by women. Men's bodies, generally speaking, all over their bodies, don't seem nearly as sensitive.

Some studies show that the amygdala in women is more active, as is the hypothalamus, which is where oxytocin is produced. Oxytocin is the love drug. For a long time, we didn't even know men produced it. We thought the only time and only place it was produced was in pregnant women and in new mothers. Now, we know that men produce plenty of it and that it's present in both during sex, and is released by the truckload at orgasm. During sex, oxytocin is just as bonding between lovers, as it is between mother and a newborn baby. Good stuff. We should bottle it and sell it in the grocery store.

Because oxytocin is associated with bonding, an emotional event, it makes sense to me that women produce more at orgasm since their orgasms are more of an emotional event than with men. That sounds like a huge generalization. But, the science backs that up. The chemistry and neurology say so.

Gay, straight, bi, trans, and virtually every type of attraction and identity, even attraction that is completely non sexual such as the feelings toward family members and plutonic friends and people you are not sexually attracted to but have feelings of love with, causes the production of oxytocin and serotonin, endorphins, and the rest of the "sex cocktail". Not as much as during orgasm, but still, enough that it can be measured.

There is no research that I have found studying the chemistry of people who have completed gender confirmation (aka gender reassignment) surgery. Between the hormones and the internal, overwhelming feeling of being born in the wrong body, I would be curious if there is any change from the CISgendered and the MISgendered. It doesn't matter in their behavior. Both are raised by the narrow two-set system. But, I would be curious how the chemistry might change from what is expected.

Anyway. The one difference that really applies to this article is that the pleasure center of a woman's brain is more easily triggered to light up than a man's brain. Not with sex. Well, of course with sex. But, all kinds of stuff triggers it!! There is an emotional stimulus that triggers it that most men don't have on the same level. Not even close. I mean, all kinds of stuff triggers a man's pleasure center. But what does it is a much smaller range of stuff, and the level that our pleasure center is triggered to light up is nowhere near that of a woman's. Basically, it takes a lot to get us men excited... About anything. Women... Well, they can get pretty excited about a whole lotta stuff.

So. With women being physically much more sensitive to pleasure and their brain working in such a way that they are "feeling it" much more than men, why are so many women not achieving orgasm the way their brains suggest that they should? I mean, according to the neurology, shouldn't women be having to pause pretty much throughout the entire day for orgasm breaks?

Just an odd fun fact. Did you know that during menstruation, the activity with the corpus callosum is the highest. Men and women, any time, ever in our entire lives, it is the highest in women who are menstruating. Literally, the left hand DOES know what the right hand is doing. Your critical analysis brain and your intuitive feeling brain are having a conversation. So, if you feel a little crazy when you're on your period, you kinda are. Jus' sayin'.

"I can't cum," says quite a few women I've talked to.

"Bullshit!" I answer. "You DON'T cum. That's different."

Why?

A few years ago, Cosmo, or some other women's magazine, did a less-than-scientific study of thousands of married women. Over 80% said they are dissatisfied with their sex life. Over 80% said that they rarely orgasm when they and their husband have sex. They gave a list of reasons. At the top of that list was that their husbands didn't take enough time and that their husbands didn't seem to know much about what makes a woman have an orgasm.

"Why the fuck did you marry him then?" I actually asked that out loud. I was sitting in a doctor's office waiting room, waiting to talk to the doctor, who was about to become a new customer of mine for my day business. Needless to say, the patients in the waiting area were not impressed with my outburst and my new customer suddenly had some reservations about our new business arrangement. We compromised for the sake of the relationship. I agreed not to read the magazines any more when I came to his office.

Anyway. Even though the article seemed like exaggerated fluff, it stuck with me. Why would so many women say that? Well, there really are reasons why those statistics might not be so exaggerated. In countless conversations I've had with women over the years, there are LOTS of women who aren't satisfied. I wouldn't say it's 80%. Although, I would say that 80% of the women I've talked to experience a lack of satisfaction more often than a full sense of satisfaction.

Why?

1) Women Are Tired

I mean… Seriously. Have you seen a woman's life? Guys, one of the best things you can do to improve your sex life is to let your woman have a nap. I say this half joking because it sounds like an odd aphrodisiac, but I'm serious. Just the stuff going on in her head would wear out most of us mere mortals.

Even in relationships where men SEEM like they are sharing things equally, "equal" has a very subjective understanding. I'm jus' sayin'. Ladies, am I right? Your man comes up behind you and starts kissing your neck. It's wonderful and all that. But, all you can think of is getting off your feet and sitting on the couch for a few. You can't though because there is still a lot to do before you can even think of switching gears. And, you're already worn out.

Such is life. It started before you were out of diapers. And now that you are married and have kids and jobs and a world on your shoulders, is it any surprise that sex isn't working the way it should?

2) Women Are Stressed

Stress is more commonly a mood killer, in men AND women, than almost any other non medical factor. If the brain is our most vital sexual organ, even more so in women, is it any surprise that when the brain is worried about other things, sex gets bumped to the back burner. Not only does it kill the mood, but it can greatly effect performance. For men, it's a major cause of ED. For women, it's a major cause of not being able to climax.

Stress doesn't magically go away when you shift gears into sex mode. It's effects on the body are still there even though you are thinking about playtime. It's on the back burner, but the things you are stressed about are still nagging you.

With most women, stress is more complicated. For men, the things stressing us out are often more easily manageable and seem to be less of a factor. Generally speaking, that is. There are also factors including self confidence that effect stress and how we process it. With women, those factors are often more complex also. The result? Putting aside stress to enjoy sex is more of a challenge.

3) Women Are Complicated

In addition to fatigue and stress, women's brains can be consumed with body image issues, self esteem issues and confidence issues. They're thinking about the relationship and how well that relationship is working. Women are more likely to have anxiety related to intimacy than men. Women are more likely to feel insecurity with a relationship.

And then there's unprocessed issues related to trauma such as sexual assault, incest and/or molestation as children, as well as all the societal influences and pressures that bombard women every single day.

All of these sound like grand generalizations about women. And I admit, they somewhat are. However, virtually every woman has some of these issues, on some level, in some combination, and to some degree. Part of it, we can blame the outdated two-set system. Part of it, we can blame evolution. And part of it, blame society. Even though we generalize these characteristics as being mostly female, ALL human beings have similar insecurities and issues. All of us. Everyone. But, these specific issues are disproportionately female in the way they effect us sexually.

Just to be clear, men have many of the same issues. All of us. Everyone. But in men, they generally manifest differently in how they effect us. And, how we process those issues is somewhat different. Bottom line, it is less likely to effect us sexually. Stress and fatigue is more likely to cause problems than our insecurities.

For 1) 2) & 3), the simple cure for all these is to take internet MEMEs more seriously. "Self Love" and "Love yourself" is actually good therapy for these things. All those sappy MEMEs are absolutely right. Show of hands. How many of you have rolled your eyes at seeing ANOTHER one of those MEMEs posted by some fit yogini eating perfectly arranged berries in paradise or some other setting that takes your breath away? (raises hand) She doesn't know your life. Fuck all that!!

The truth is though, it's true. Stop rolling your eyes. Self love takes many, many forms and it begins with tiny little steps. Even small steps have a great benefit. Any time people step in a positive direction, it snowballs. Positive choices lead to more positive choices just as negative choices lead to more negative choices. As silly as some of those MEMEs are, find some small steps towards loving yourself better and you'll see that they aren't so silly.

All that self love and taking care of yourself, works. From dealing with a little insecurity to making progress on major issues, the work begins in small ways that are almost unnoticeable. They compound. Like going to the gym one time won't drop your weight, going to the gym regularly will. Small changes in how we think and how we look at things will add up to results that aren't so small. The most apparent result is that our sex life gets better.

Those are the least complicated issues for why you don't cum. Let's dig deeper.

4) Men Need To Change What They're Learning

In an informal survey with other sexologist I talk to, as well as some that I don't talk to very often, men ask for advice less than 10% of the total number of people asking for advice. I have been asking this question for about 5 years and my personal survey group consist of only about 100 people. Seemingly, a very small set to draw a conclusion from. But, considering that each of those people, including myself, has talked to thousands of people, that study set isn't as small as it initially seems.

Before assembling this piece, I went back through the last 100 conversations I have had. Out of that 100, only 2 were from men. So, I went back further. I went back to January 1st, 2018 to all the conversations I have had where someone asked me for suggestions or information. Altogether, I have had 1,506 conversations. Only 8 were conversations with men. That's about .005%

I went back to the group and asked, "If men aren't asking for help, where do you think they are gathering information from?" The general consensus is that SOME men are doing their own homework. This is awesome!! There are LOTS of men out there that are knowledgeable and educated on sex. Some, I dare say, know even more than I do on some topics. So, just because they aren't asking experts, doesn't mean that men aren't learning.

Women seem to be more open minded to learning from others. Consider the 2-set system of conditioning. Women are more inclined to value learning from others directly through their relationship with that person. Men are taught to be independent. And independently, some men ARE learning stuff.

Sooooo.... Why do so many women complain that their men don't know anything? Could it really be as high as 80% of women who think that? Maybe. Maybe not.

Guys, work on the way things FEEL before you start trying to make her feel good physically. SLOW THINGS DOWN. Instead of beginning with, "Let's have sex," and then initiating your five-minute plan that ends with you shooting your load into her and falling asleep, try a slower plan. Just a suggestion.

She's going to need more time to switch gears from life to pleasure.

I know. That is such a bad stereotype of how men define sex with their wives and girlfriends. I'd like to think it isn't like that most of the time and in most relationships. I would LOVE to think otherwise. However, I cannot count the number of conversations I have had with women, men and couples where this horrible stereotype is all too common.

5) Conditioning

The biggest reasons are bigger. It has to do with that two-set system that almost every single one of us is trained to fit into from the day we are born. Naturally, we work a certain way. Men work the way they work and women work they way they work, both in very predictable ways based on the way we were conditioned to experience the world long before we ever thought about sex. Gay, straight, bi, trans, queer, non binary, non conforming, all of us, with few exceptions. Generally speaking, this is how we are. Blame the world. Blame evolution somewhat too, but mostly blame the world. Our brains work slightly different from each other. True. But the real reason is that we were trained to be the way we are.

Gay men. You can be fem and pretty, and FABULOUS. But, I'll bet you still work just like straight guys most of the time and in most ways. Gay women too. When it comes to sex, we may have a wide range of individuality. But, HOW we process the experience of sex in our brains still fits the same binary system. I know there are exceptions to every rule and if you believe you are the exception, I'm fine with that.

We are trained from day one to have very traditional roles and function according to those roles. No matter how we grow and change and evolve over the course of our lives, that training sticks with us in the back of our brains like a default setting. As different as we all become, we are all very much alike.

I'm not man-bashing. I'm really not. Many men are wonderful and justify the continued interest in them. What I'm bashing is our limited programming that we are all conditioned with that tilts everything in our bedrooms.

In many ways, women have strayed from the things that actually get them off. It's a man's world. A man probably pushed you to have sex the first time. A man took control of what you did and when and where and you ADAPTED to him. You might enjoy porn. You might enjoy some of the "weird stuff" he likes and maybe some "weird stuff" of your own. You might be very goal-oriented when you have sex. But, you might also be just as happy enjoying the journey with no specific goal in mind. This seems to work well if your man is your Dom and you are his sub... Until it doesn't.

And just to be clear, I am not saying there is anything wrong with traditional gender roles. Many families that I've talked to fall into those roles. Maybe even most of them. It works for them. If it works for you, then don't fix it if it ain't broke. Traditional gender roles are simpler and easier because that's how society trained us to be. For many relationships, those roles work just fine.

Remember though, all that old fashioned stuff shamed women for their sexuality and wasn't exactly female friendly for most of history. A woman enjoying her "wifely duties"? NO WAY!! A woman wanting to enjoy sex? Shameful hussey!! Whore! Slut! Words of endearment, now, when spoken by your favorite someone. But, for most of recorded history they were NOT the words you wanted to hear.

When you were younger, things seemed so much simpler. Everything was fun. Everything seemed to work better. Now, there are kids and you just got divorced and there is a job you're not thrilled with and homework and men that aren't interested - or worse, aren't worth you being interested in them. And when you finally find someone "sponge-worthy" (if you remember that reference from Seinfeld), you aren't reaching the happy ending. Why are you surprised?

"I don't know why I can't cum."

Not calling Anorgasmia a myth, but, "No. You DON'T cum.That's different."

BTW. Anorgasmia is a real condition that effects some women. I don't know what the most common cause is according to the medical community. But in MY experience with the women I've talked to, it is usually medication or hormones that causes it. That is a whole different situation from this. See the first part of this series.

"My husband does everything right. It used to work and I'd cum fine. Now, it doesn't work."

Yep. That's what I'm talking about. If it's not the hormones. And, it's not the meds. And, you got plenty of rest and you don't have a health issue and you're not worried about the kids and everything else that MIGHT be causing the problem, now we can get down to the real reason this is a problem.

All that old fashioned conditioning is finally taking it's toll on your amygdala.

Part 3:
First Contact

Let me talk about first times. I'm fascinated by the stories women tell me about their first time to experience an orgasm. Nothing surprises me anymore. Well, if a woman told me that everything went according to script, that would surprise me. Meet someone, develop a nice relationship, they have sex and orgasms flow as natural as a mountain stream. Really? Has that EVER happened for ANY woman?

I put sexual development into four stages, at least in the context of this discussion. If a child is sexualized in some way outside the norm, either through molestation or some other event, these stages can get twisted up all over the map. But, without such an event, this is the basics of natural development.

First contact is when the questions begin and the hormones start their reign in the body. It is when young people begin masturbating and exploring their bodies. I call it "contact" because they are "contacting" their sexual self and making the connection to the person they are internally. I have always believed that our sexuality is the core of who/how/what we are as human beings. It is connection to that sexual self that brings us peace and self acceptance.

Second contact is when we bring all that naivety and ignorance into our relationships with other people. This stage starts when we start talking to our friends, or maybe our parents. It continues through the first time you let a boy get to "second base". It continues through losing your virginity, and all those first sexual experiences that are usually less than memorable.

Third contact is when things start to get interesting. First orgasm with a partner. First time trying some new things. First time having types of sex and sex in situations other than the narrow definition of "normal" that we are fed by the world around us as we are growing up.

Fourth contact is when things go from "interesting" to "HOLY FUCK!! WHAT WAS THAT? AND PLEEEEEEASE DO IT AGAIN!!" This is when things all come together and result in full discovery of the sexual self. Call it nirvana. Call it enlightenment. Call it fully balancing your chakras. Call it whatever you like, but it's when everything starts making sense and your wonderful journey of sexuality REALLY begins.

Of the thousands of conversations I have had with women, and the thousands of cases I have read by other people, I am blown away at the number of people who never reached third contact. Women AND men. They have sex because it feels good and it's the expected behavior of people in a relationship. But sadly, it never really gets interesting.

Even sadder, the number of people who reach fourth contact is a very, very small percentage.

Janice had her first orgasm when she was 15. She had played with her vagina for about 6 months. She had even experimented with fingering her ass because a girl at school had talked to her about anal sex. "Can't get pregnant from anal", she said. And there were a couple of girls that were doing that with their boyfriends. Vagina and anus felt nice, but didn't do anything special.

One night, she was massaging her newly developed breasts and it happened. She told me that she even lactated a little and suddenly it all made sense to her. For years, she thought that was how it worked for other girls. She was in college before she had an orgasm from anything else, even masturbating. She never knew.

What kinda depressed me about her story was that after it happened, she worked up her courage and told to her mom about it. Her mom didn't believe her. She said that never happened. And when Janice insisted that it did, her mom took her to the doctor to make sure there wasn't something wrong with her.

Luckily, the doctor let her know she was just fine and gave her a little bit of a human sexuality lesson. Her mother never did believe that it happened that way. Janet thinks it's possible that her mother had never experienced an orgasm. We'll never know because Janice's mom would never talk about sex in any way.

Now, happily married in her 40s to a guy that sounds like a wonderfully adventurous lover, Janice has ALL KINDS of orgasms from applying what happened with her breasts to other parts of her body. That's how she learned to have clitoral orgasms and all the others she has now. She even learned how to achieve psycholagny simply with recall of what she had done with her breasts.

Klara was 22 when she had her first orgasm. She was raised in a very religious home and was shamed against masturbating. She was even told that she would "Burn in Hell" for it. So, she had never explored her own body in any way.

Not only was she not a virgin, she was the mother of a 2 year old. One night after sex with her husband, she went to pee. When she wiped herself off, it happened out of nowhere. After she collected herself, she went back in the bedroom and told her husband, "Play with THIS and see what happens." She had no idea about her own body. Knew nothing and neither did her husband.

Her husband, who, like her, secretly wasn't as religious as they had to maintain appearances of. They began to learn about their bodies and experiment with sex. Eventually, they left the church. And now, as members of a more open-minded religious fellowship, they teach others to go learn. They work with couples in their church to improve their sex lives, improve intimacy through education, and develop a better marriage through that intimate adventure.

Another woman, Janet, had her first orgasm when she was 28. She had 3 kids from 3 different boyfriends and hadn't been to a GYN since her last child was born 4 years earlier. Her family had lived in poverty her entire life. She was the first person in her family to graduate high school. Alcoholism or drugs or abuse wasn't a problem in her family, like many in that position. They just had a history of poverty and a lack of education.

One day, she was trying on jeans in Walmart. She had finally lost the weight she had gained during her last pregnancy and was shopping for some skinny jeans. When she pulled them up, they were tight!! She had, as she described it, "an absolutely EPIC camel toe". Nothing seemed to straighten things out. And, the more she tried to get rid of the camel toe, the more aroused she got.

Next thing you know, she had to sit down on the bench in the little changing room. Her first orgasm made it impossible to stand up. She thinks she even squealed a little. Flushed, sweating, out of breath, she had to get it together to leave the changing room because her friend was standing there with her kids.

She went home and began experimenting and managed to learn how to bring herself to orgasm without the tight jeans. It was almost 10 years before she told anyone about that. It was 12 years before she was able to duplicate the magic with a lover.

Nat, short for Natalie, had her first orgasm at 37. After her husband left her for the secretary, leaving her with 3 kids and a 15 year old Toyota, she didn't even date for a couple of years. She had a male coworker that she became friends with. She liked him, but didn't, you know, "like him like him". He was fun to have coffee with, but she didn't want it to go any further.

One night, he was over at her apartment having dinner with her and the kids. After dinner, he helped her clean up. And then he helped her get the kids to bed. And then they opened a bottle of wine. A couple glasses later, the coworker confessed that he was hoping they could take their relationship a little deeper.

At first, that raised every red flag in Nat's brain and she almost threw him out. But then, she thought, 'Sooner or later, I have to get back on the horse.' He was a decent guy. He was good with her and good with her kids. So, why not?

It turns out, he's a decent guy in bed too. Patient and fun, much more knowledgeable than her husband had been, he gave her several orgasms that night and it was a life changing event. They have been together now over 10 years on their way to forever. They never married and they're both okay with that.

Theresa had all kind of orgasms when she was a teenager and exploring her own body. She had orgasms penetrating herself with her fingers and random household objects. She had orgasms playing with her clit. She had them from fingering her ass. She even had some nice orgasms from her fingers in her mouth and touching her lips.

Immediately after high school, she married her sweetheart and had sex for the first time. It was terrible. There were no orgasms and her husband was such a prude that he wasn't willing to do anything to get her there. Then came the kids. Then came all the pressure for her to stay in the marriage from family, friends and their church. Next thing she knew, over 20 years had gone by and she forgot all about pleasure.

Then the kids moved out and went to college and were living their own lives. And suddenly, she had some time to explore. She and her husband had separate lives that barely intersected. With the kids gone, there was all this time for her to fill. She remembered how she spent a lot of time as a teenager and decided that would be a fun new hobby.

At first, there were no orgasms. She had hit menopause and her hormones weren't cooperating. And, there was a learning curve, physically, mentally, emotionally and spiritually. She had changed considerably physically, mentally, emotionally and spiritually. After all that time, she had to relearn how to give herself pleasure. Even though she tried almost daily, it took her almost a year before she had her next orgasm.

Flora had her first orgasm at 44. Her mother never told her anything about sex. Her mother never told her much of anything. Flora was 4x divorced with 5 grown kids and had just never learned anything about how it should work.

One night, a friend dragged her to a "toy party". And when she resisted even touching the toys, her friend bought her a vibrator anyway. And when they got back home, she basically held her down and used it on her. At first, that sounds like lesbian rape, but Flora assured me it wasn't like that. Neither woman was a lesbian. But her friend cared enough about her deprived friend to cross that bridge. Flora is still grateful.

I dated a woman that I have referred to as Sunshine in other writings. You'll have to go read about her. A shocking story in some ways. She was 48 and had never been wet before. You heard me. Well, she admitted that maybe she had, she just wasn't aware of it. When we kissed for the first time, she became aware that she got very wet and actually thought her cooter was busted. She asked her friend about it and had to be convinced that she was fine.

Along with complete unawareness about getting wet being a natural process, she had been convinced by her first husband that the female orgasm was a myth. You heard me. A myth!! Like, an urban legend. Like Bigfoot. Really. That's how he mansplained it to her.

So you can imagine what I thought. I saw it as my personal mission to educate her. I wanted to teach her everything!! Sadly, the relationship didn't go very well. We dated for quite a while, but it was very on and off. Intimacy totally freaked her out. She had given herself so fully to her ex husband and for it to fail after over 25 years together, the very concepts of trust and vulnerability and connection in healthy ways, made her run for the hills.

She was actually a much more intelligent woman than this probably suggest about her. But, she grew up in ignorance and got married right after high school and her husband kept her in ignorance. Very intelligent!! But the people around her perpetuated a level of ignorance that is staggering. I'll have to share the story about her. It's very interesting, and funny.

Her first orgasm was with my fingers. We were kissing and my hand was working on her clit. When she got close, she actually tried to wrestle away from me because it freaked her out so much. Her second orgasm was with my mouth. That freaked her out even more. Eventually, she had orgasms from anal sex and even a few throatgasms. A couple of times, I think she maybe had a nipplegasm. But, she was so freaked out by that that she never said anything.

Lucky for her, she quickly got past the ignorance and went on a wonderful adventure. I introduced her to toys of every kind and after some serious convincing, she learned to masturbate regularly. Imagine being almost 50 and that was where your sexuality was. I don't miss her fear. But, I kinda miss seeing the look in her eyes when she learned something new.

The majority of women tell me that, at some point, as teenagers, they started exploring their bodies and discovered a happy accident. That's awesome. I think that's probably how it SHOULD happen. But from there, it is still very learned to be able to make it happen whenever they want, and there's even more learning to make it happen with a partner. The learning curve is steep.

One of the things that does surprise me is the number of women in their 40s and beyond who have never had an orgasm of any kind from any type of stimulation. I am even more surprised at how many women in their 40s know NOTHING about their own anatomy or how it all works. "I THINK I had one once, but I'm not sure." Lady, I'm thinking if you had one, you'd be sure.

How is this possible? How is it that we have such a society that makes this possible? Religious beliefs and an absolutely ignorant society drowning in ancient social standards is how. It just seems that somehow we would have gained some ground somewhere in this.

"Tradition" is peer pressure from a bunch of dead people. Jus' sayin'.

Sexuality is the least financed of all types of research, with female sexuality being the worst of all. It's improving in the last 10 years or so. But, we are in the 21st century, people!! This is so wrong!!

People want to project an image that we are all polite society and never do those kinds of things. Yet, everywhere we look, people are having sex. Many of them, sex that is outside the narrow, vanilla definition of "normal". We KNOW that we're all having sex. Why are we such prudes when virtually every person on the planet is getting their freak on in some way??? Why can't we talk about it, study it, learn about it, and BE HEALTHY with it?????????

If I accomplish only one thing in my life, it will be to encourage women to not settle for bad sex. They'll have to drag the men kicking and screaming because most men are slow to warm to making things better in the bedroom. They will have to overcome thousands of years of societal repression and unease with public discussion of intimate topics. But, if we can all get a little more open to learning, we can fix this. Sadly though, I suspect it will likely take another thousand years. (heavy sigh)

Part 4:
Dirty Thoughts

These are just some random thoughts that are kinda related. They are in no particular order. Just some thoughts I collected in putting this series together and I wasn't sure where to fit them in otherwise.

"Feminism isn't about making women strong. Women are already strong. It's about changing the way the world perceives that strength." ~ G. D. Anderson

Barry Komisaruk, who is a psychologist at Rutgers, and one of my personal heroes, along with Beverly Whipple, has done some amazing work on orgasms with women who have suffered spinal cord injuries. One of their discoveries is that it is very possible to create new neurological pathways, or utilize alternate pathways, such as the vagus nerve and completely remap the senses to get there. It's all a matter of learning. You might not consider sex to be essential to human existence, but the brain does. Especially in women.

Think about the way that you and your man have sex. Men control everything in the bedroom. They decide what you're doing and how you're doing it. That has to change if you want things to change. Men, for the most part, are not the ones who are dissatisfied. Men, for the most part, are getting their orgasms. There is little motivation for them to change things if women don't demand better. Not to blame the victim (much), but women will have to initiate change or it is unlikely to happen.

For men, sex is primary a physical event. For women, it is cerebral and emotional, and THEN physical. The best sex you'll ever have is when these things are merged better between you and your man.

There are countless people on the internet screaming about this divide. They are teaching classes, offering videos and books and tools. Resources are out there. If you aren't willing to invest some time and maybe a little money in things getting better, they won't get better.

5 things women wish men would do:
1) Make eye contact
2) Slow down!!
3) Use your hands and fingers all over
4) Communicate that you are enjoying yourself. Let her know!! Be more vocal.
5) Ask questions. Don't be so arrogant to think you know everything about ANY partner.

During sex, men worry about performance, women worry about appearance. Men feel anxiety about their performance, women feel anxiety about their bodies.

When there is greater joy in the rest of your life, the greater the pleasure in your sex life. It takes the pressure off your partner to "give" you pleasure. And, it takes the pressure off you to perform. When you are alive, it shows in your sexual energy. You can't be a half for a whole relationship. Only two whole people can do that.

Many aspects of sex trigger feelings of shame or embarrassment, even some guilt. You should not feel guilt or shame or embarrassment about having a sex life that feels natural to you. If you do feel those things, start there. When those things are resolved, your sex life will get infinitely better.

Organic shame makes us feel bad about out behavior. We do something we believe is wrong. That is natural. It says we are human and have some sense of morality. Implanted shame makes us feel bad about ourselves. That is not natural. Organic shame: I did something wrong. Implanted shame: There's something wrong with me.

Emotions are embedded deep in the subconscious by the limbic system. Locked into memory and they come up at the oddest times. Usually when you're THIS CLOSE to having an orgasm. That is when all the emotions in your head are firing on all cylinders. And thus, that is how all the crap in your head prevents you from having an orgasm.

It is also how women can remember, verbatim, what you said in an argument 5 years ago. Arguing is also an emotional event for women. So, the memory of that argument is embedded a lot more securely than all the stuff a man remembers.

So, if some lover in her past told her something negative at an emotional moment, like, during sex, it stuck there and it is a bitch to get rid of.

Men, if you want to remember things better, use the same method. Make them emotional in some way. How you do that is up to you. I'm a man. I have no suggestions for achieving it. Just kidding. Actually, hold your wife's hand while you argue and you'll be on a level playing field. The two of you are also more likely to resolve the argument sooner and with less bloodshed.

Stop comparing yourself to pornstars and what you see in porn. AND, stop letting your lovers compare you to porn. As human beings, NONE of us live up to the fantasy. The irony is that when you stop comparing yourself to what you see in the video, you can actually experience sex that is way beyond that.

Many women say that working on their sexuality feels like work. It's exhausting. If the one thing that brings pleasure feels like work, no wonder more women aren't feeling pleasure.

Most sex education is all wrong. Men receive almost none and what women receive is mostly negative.

There's nothing wrong with you or your body. Your body is doing exactly what it is comfortable with, even when it doesn't make sense. You have to feel safe enough to be vulnerable to let go. If you can't let go, look at what ways you are not feeling mentally and emotionally comfortable. Take small steps towards finding emotional comfort, even if those steps don't make sense at first.

I had a girlfriend that was bothered by the ceiling fan. It triggered a negative memory that she couldn't let go of.

A woman in a study I read about was bothered by a clock that chimed at all the wrong times. When it chimed, it was like it was telling her, "Time's up!" and she would be suddenly, completely not in the mood any more. Her boyfriend would get her aroused all over again, and then the clock would chime. They got rid of the clock and had wonderful sex.

A man I talked to noticed that his wife wouldn't orgasm before 9:00 pm. But at 9:01, she could cum like crazy. That was the kids' bedtime. Before that, she was nervous about the kids interrupting them. After 9:00, she was no longer worried about it.

If you can't cum, look at the negative messages that are festering in the back of your brain. Just as the world gets more and more sexualized, the world seems to get more and more judgmental and negative about individual sexuality. We are surrounded by toxic statements and messages. Many are ridiculous and we don't actually believe them. But, how many of those ridiculous statements are floating around in your brain when you are trying to have an orgasm?

"…quick fix, genital sneeze solution for orgasm…"

LMAO!!!!!!!! I don't know where I heard that and in what context, or if it's a note I wrote down somewhere. Maybe I read it somewhere. I don't remember. In the thousands of notes doing the research for this series, I wrote that down. Wherever it came from, it's important. Maybe one of us will remember it when we need it most and it will make perfect sense. In the meantime, it makes absolutely no sense to me. It just makes me laugh.

Part 5: Faking It

One of the most discouraging conversations I have had with women is about faking orgasms. I realize all the reasons that women do it. But, don't do that!! Stop faking orgasms!! It does not make things better.

Here are the most common reasons I have heard for why women fake orgasms:

"I'm done. I just want this to be over."

Some women fake them because they want the sex to be over. Either they have given up on having an orgasm or they know it isn't possible with what their lover is doing to/for/with them. After some time, they have lost interest in the sex and just want it to be over without hurting their lover's feelings. So, they fake an orgasm hoping that will be the end of things.

Sometimes, she didn't want to have sex at all, so she fakes an orgasm to hurry up and be done with it. This is common in domestic violence situations.

"He'll be mad at ME if he thinks I didn't orgasm."

She doesn't want to upset her lover. As long as he/she thinks they are getting her off, everything is fine. This one was also common among women who were victims of domestic violence. A woman told me that she didn't have an orgasm when her boyfriend raped her in the car after she bailed him out of jail for beating up his OTHER girlfriend. So, he beat her up, half naked, in the car, in the parking of the police station. After that, she faked it every time to avoid getting beat up.

"All my other girlfriends had plenty of orgasms. It's not MY fault. There must be something wrong with YOU."

If a lover shames her enough times, it's easy to start believing that it really is the woman's fault. To avoid that, she fakes it. He must be right. Right?

There is also the possibility that it began with a lack of knowing anything and it snowballed from there. As a teenager beginning to explore sex, healthy information is in short supply. So when a young woman doesn't know how it works, and her only source of feedback is the guy she's with, who also doesn't know much, it's very easy for this ignorance to become engrained. Ignorance begets more ignorance.

"I don't know how it all works. If I keep faking it, eventually, I'll figure it out."

Some women fake orgasms because they are inexperienced and have possibly never had one. Or, they haven't had them regularly and don't know how to make them happen. It is possible they are embarrassed and don't want their lover to think they are incompetent and don't know how to orgasm. They fake it, hoping it will eventually happen and they won't have to fake it anymore.

"There MUST be something wrong with ME. That's not my lover's fault. I don't want him/her to feel bad."

So, she fakes it.

"Oh, it's okay. I don't need an orgasm to be happy with our sex life."

Some women are reluctant to receive pleasure. It's like they think they don't deserve it. Or, some women are complete givers and for sex to be an equally enjoyed activity is awkward for them. They have learned how to be the giver and they know the role well. But, receiving pleasure is unknown territory and so uncomfortable that they avoid it altogether.

"Orgasm? That's really personal and private. I'm not comfortable sharing that with someone."

It could be that she is embarrassed to orgasm with someone. In many cases, that is a trust issue and/or an issue with being vulnerable with their partner. To let go of control requires more trust than she has for the person. So, she fakes it. Somehow pretending to orgasm is okay but letting go and having one isn't.

"When I let go, I make this crazy, yelling noise and shake all over. Nobody wants to see that."

It's possible she is embarrassed about her orgasm behavior when she loses control. So, she manufactures sounds or behavior that is less embarrassing. Or something she saw in a movie. One woman said she spied on a friend having sex with her boyfriend and she made a cute little noise and did "this thing" and it was cute. So, she mimicked her friend for years. THEN, years later, she found out that her friend was faking it.

"Oh, my orgasms aren't anything to brag about."

On the opposite end, a few women have told me that even their best orgasms DID NOT elicit wild noises and body thrashing and a complete loss of control. Great orgasms, just not what they thought that should look like. They thought they were boring. Or, they thought there was something wrong with them. Sooooo... They may have had a wonderful orgasm but faked the behavior that went along with it.

"If I don't have spectacular orgasms, he'll leave me."

The wild fake orgasms made their husbands and lovers think they were sex gods and it insured they would never leave them. The women that told me that were all divorced. Their husbands left them.

Sigh.

In my perfect world, everyone is having great sex and they're with a partner that is perfect for them. Ugh!! Wouldn't that be wonderful? Well, we all know it isn't a perfect world. There are many, many reasons that women fake orgasms to compensate for the world's imperfections.

But faking orgasms, for whatever reason, as necessary as it seems, is not an answer.

First, it's dishonest.

If you are happy, in a healthy relationship you want to continue, an open, honest dialogue about sex is vital. If he/she is a keeper, they'll listen. They will WANT to please you and they will want to find ways that work for you too. As embarrassing as it might be, once you start, it might build intimacy and bond you with your partner even more. Imagine what a great journey the two of you can go on!! To continue faking it guarantees that your journey is going nowhere.

If you aren't getting your needs met and you don't communicate that, you are accepting it as is. Any work, whatever that may be, will never happen. You can't hope it will get better if you don't begin by voicing the problem. For many women I've talked to, this is incredibly difficult. But beginning the conversation is a must or nothing changes.

Second, it says that your pleasure isn't important or that YOU aren't important.

A phazillion social media memes will disagree. YOU are important. Your pleasure is important. And if you aren't feeling that, change is in order. It's easy for me to say that from this side of the computer screen. I know from the women I have worked with that the work is not easy and it takes fucking forever. But I have never talked to a single woman - not one - who regrets making the changes and doing the work to feel better and enjoy life more.

The first thing necessary is deciding that you want it to be better MORE than you want it to stay the same. Until you do, you won't be consistent with the work or the changes. You also have to believe it. That's something you CAN fake it until you make it. You might not feel it right away. It might take some serious faking it at first. But if you begin the journey, you'll see the results. It WILL get better.

Third, in some cases, the relationship must change.

I know, also easier said than done. From working with domestic violence victims, I know that there are a thousand reasons that women don't leave a relationship. You have to decide you're worth something better and have confidence that if you leave, things will work out. Staying where you are isn't a requirement. Once you do, there are resources available. Nothing changes until it does.

Even if there is no violence, a relationship where you aren't valued and your pleasure isn't valued is a relationship that needs to change. Some relationships are worth the work. Some aren't. There's nothing wrong with making a decision about that. I am not suggesting anyone to abandon a relationship that they are happy in. I am only saying that you have to decide if the relationship has a chance of getting better if you AND your partner do the work. If it doesn't, you need an exit strategy.

Last, faking an orgasm isn't usually the most serious thing in a relationship. But, your pleasure is important and you have to feel worthy of it. Eventually, it WILL impact your relationship. As long as your partner doesn't know, you are putting a wall up that prevents complete intimacy. In most cases, some open, honest conversation will resolve the whole thing. If you need help talking to your partner, I suggest you find a professional. There's nothing wrong with that. If that's not an option, check with other resources in your area.

I asked about a dozen women that I have worked with over the past 10 years or so, "How often do you fake an orgasm?"

Many told me that as they matured, they faked them less and less, and usually don't anymore. Many told me that as they got more experienced with sex, they faked them less and less, and usually don't anymore. Many told me that their relationship had to change, and others told me that they had to change relationships. After that, they faked them less and less, and usually don't anymore. Some told me that BEFORE, they were faking it as much as 100% of the time and they never had an orgasm with their lover.

My second question was, "Do you orgasm every time now?" Every one of them laughed and told me they don't, but almost never feel the need to fake it. Either they are comfortable enough with their sexuality that it's okay if it doesn't happen every time. Or sometimes, they are having sex that is less goal oriented. Most told me that as they matured, they chose their lovers better and now, neither they nor their lover is going to get too upset if everything doesn't go perfect. The irony of that is that when the pressure is off, things go perfect a lot more often.

The bottom line is the one I am always going on and on about. I want everyone to be having great sex. Sex is linked to every single thing about us directly or indirectly. To me, faking orgasms is a sign that some things need to change. It doesn't have to be perfect - in fact, great sex rarely is. But it needs to be real, and it needs to be real honest for it to ever be great.

Part 6:
Faking It Addendum

After I so proudly posted my series "Why Can't I Cum?", which included a section about faking orgasms, I was contacted by a woman named Karina. Did I say, "proudly"? I was. Seriously. I thought it was a very good series and had a lot of good information. As always, I just want to help people have great sex and I thought the series was a good one for that goal.

Karina reminded me of our play sessions, which were totally off script when it comes to faking orgasms. So, I am adding a small addendum to cover a different side of this issue.

See, once a good connection is developed between lovers, your lover should be able to tell when a woman fakes it. He (used generically), should be able to tell the difference between a real orgasm and a fake one.

Every woman has a "tell" when she fakes it. It's usually subtle if she's used to faking them. But subtle as it may be, it's there. Sadly, many men never notice. Sadly-er, many women know that their man won't know the difference. Sadly-est, this is okay with both of them.

For me, it's not okay. I NEVER want a woman to feel the need to fake an orgasm with me. I'm okay with things not working perfect and if we BOTH had a good time, I can live with that imperfection. But, if the problem is something I'm not doing or that I'm not doing right, I can work on that. And, I try to be comfortable and easy to talk to so she can give me the instructions I'm missing. If I am not giving her a safe space to express herself, to me, that is even worse than failing at any sexual techniques.

For me, it really isn't about whether I made her cum or not. Of course, I want her t cum 100 times every time we're together. But more important, I want her to feel freedom. I want to be the kind of man that doesn't put pressure on her to perform. That kind of pressure makes her satisfaction about ME, not HER. That's backwards.

In some cases, it's not me. It's her. She's not comfortable letting go yet if our relationship is new or if there is something else that is holding her back. I'm patient and know if I keep being a decent guy, it'll happen when she's ready. No pressure. Focus on the fun we're having and let things happen in their own time.

And then there's Karina.

We met about 20 years ago. We hit it off right away and even over coffee, we knew that sex was inevitable. She bragged that she was the most orgasmic woman I'd ever meet. I told her she'd have to prove that because, not to brag, women tend to be very orgasmic with me. I know stuff and I have skills. Jus' sayin'.

When the inevitable happened the first time, she just melted in my arms when we were kissing. I've never thought I was a great kisser, but it seemed to really work on her. All our clothes were still on and she seemed like she had something happening. And as the clothes came off and I was kissing her body, she seemed to have more urgent stuff happening. I considered, for a moment, that she might actually prove what she claimed.

The "trick", for me, depends on giving a woman a REAL orgasm. If I don't, she might actually be able to fool me temporarily. There are clues that divide real from fake. Breathing is one. Reflexive body responses are a good one, too. Some things can't be faked if you know what you're looking for.

Once she has a REAL orgasm, basing that on what I know can't be faked, I will immediately recognize the tells. If a man - any man - pays extra close attention, he can recognize them too.

Best I could tell, Karina had about 50 orgasms that night over a 3 hour span. Only 3 or 4 were real though. In her case, when she had a real orgasm, she needed a moment for the sensitivity to taper off before I could continue. Her breathing changed too. She tried to fake that. But with the fake ones, she missed the little hitch at the peak where she completely stopped breathing for a second. The fake ones, she didn't have that entirely. She was probably not even aware of what EXACTLY happened when she really had an orgasm.

At some point, instead of getting upset, or losing interest, I decided I was going to have some fun with her. Some of my best skills are not with sex, but with mischief. If she was going to play it this way, I was going to teach her a lesson.

I didn't tell her that night. I agreed with her that she was very impressive. But, I also held back and arrogantly told her that she didn't really impress ME too much. After all, I'm the guy with skills and experience. I went on to tell her that my ex, who ironically had introduced us, orgasmed like that regularly and it just wasn't a big deal.

As we cuddled in the afterglow and I told her that, she gave me a "challenge accepted" look. That was exactly what I was hoping for. Hehehe!!

A few nights later, we went on a vanilla date. I took her to a Smokies game. She faked one while she ate a hotdog in a VERY inappropriate way with all the people around us watching, like the scene in "When Harry met Sally.". I think she was trying to tell me that she has orgasms when she gives head. I had told her that was one of my absolute favorite things and I think she was hoping that I would like her more if she did that. I'm just guessing.

Later, in the car, she went down on me for a little bit while we waited for traffic to clear out. She faked a couple of orgasms. But by this time, I could tell. I played it up though. I repeatedly told her how much I love that and how special that made her to me. I told her that the ex never came from giving me head, as much as I wanted it to happen.

Her reply? That she LOVED having orgasms that way. They were some of the best and it was one of her favorite ways to orgasm.

I was in.

The next time we were together, I did all the things that would cause her to FAKE an orgasm and none of the things that had actually given her a REAL one. And each time she seemed like she was getting close to a real one, I put my dick in her mouth, which would take her over the edge of several fake orgasms.

No real orgasms though. Lots and lots of fake ones, but no real ones.

The next time we were together, I mostly had my dick in her mouth and not much else. She faked some orgasms in spectacular fashion. But I began to notice a new tell. She was losing interest in the stuff that led to a fake orgasm.

Twice more, we had a similar evening. A whole evening with no real orgasms for her in spite of some wonderful playing. I had fun. Her, not so much.

The time after that, she realized that I had been playing with her. In the middle of her faking one, I snickered a little. I couldn't help it.

She flopped on the bed and asked how long I had known. I told her, "From the first night we were together."

She was genuinely hurt. "Why didn't you tell me?"

"Why didn't you tell me you'd rather fake orgasms than have real ones?"

"You're mean," she mumbled and started to tear up.

"You could have had all the REAL orgasms that you wanted. You made a choice. All you had to do was be honest with me."

Then the crying started. The lip quivering. The tears. She was good. Breathing gave it away though. "You can't even cry honestly, can you?"

Instantly, the crying changed to anger. She was busted and she knew it. I've never seen a woman get dressed that fast and hit the door. I've earned some fast exits before, but never one like that.

Within an hour, the ex was on the phone. Karina had told her everything. The ex was laughing so hard she couldn't make full sentences. Through several conversations back and forth, everyone found some peace (and a few laughs). Karina learned her lesson and swore she would never fake an orgasm again.

I don't know if that's true. I never talked to Karina again until she called about the article. The ex and I stayed friends for a couple of years and she mentioned Karina every once in a while. I asked if she was holding up her promise. "Well, except when I NEED to fake one." Apparently she likes that sometimes.

Bottom line. There is no need to fake an orgasm. I understand all the reasons why women do. But, there is no need to EVER fake an orgasm. If you lover is paying attention, they'll eventually figure it out. When they do, it will end badly. Jus' sayin'. If you're in a relationship or situation where you are not free to orgasm OR NOT orgasm, that is definitely the first step that must be resolved.

Part 7:
Vibrator Dependency

Vibrators are awesome, ain't they? Of all the crazy things human beings have invented. I put vibrators in the top ten. They're right up there with the wheel, computers, the electric guitar, cable TV, indoor plumbing and those thingees that launch a tennis ball for the dog to chase.

You probably didn't read this about me. I kinda buried it in another story. But back in the 80s, I actually invented a particular type of vibrator. You know the one with the little beads in it? You're welcome.

Anyway. Vibrators are really great… Until they're not. And by "not", I mean that point where it's the only way a woman can orgasm.

It's really not fair. No lover can match what a vibrator can do. The sensations are so intense and incredible. I mean, seriously, does it get any better than that? A lover can't compete. Not even close.

I talked to a woman recently, Gina, who admitted that she spent her entire tax refund check 3 years in a row on vibrators. She had every kind there is. Some, she bought a few of them in case one breaks. She hadn't been with a man in almost 7 years. Didn't need one anymore. As long as she could hire one to cut the grass and fix the car, she didn't have any need for a man. Her vibrators were all she would ever need.

In a goal-oriented, over sexualized culture that says orgasm is the reason we exist, a good vibrator is an easy way to knock one out quickly and efficiently. When all else has failed to deliver, a vibrator restores a woman's confidence that there is nothing wrong and she can have as many orgasms as she wants in the time allowed. Nothing wrong with that. Right?

Weeeeelllll… Yes, there is.

First thing, let me go over how an orgasm works. You know it doesn't actually happen in the body, don't you? Nope. It happens in the brain. It is the release of chemicals into the system that gives you the euphoria, not whatever happened with the body that led you there. It is an almost automatic cause and effect situation. Do THIS to the body, the brain responds with what it believes is the appropriate action.

Sex consists of two separate parts. First, there is the activity with the body. The "cause". Like a default setting, the brain has learned that certain things should trigger orgasm as the appropriate response. And when the body is engaged in an activity that the brain has associated as causing orgasm, it releases a wonderful chemical cocktail into our system and we feel amazing. That cocktail has lots and lots of dopamine, oxytocin, serotonin, vasopressin, melatonin, a little nitric oxide and finishes off with some prolactin to help you sleep better.

For the majority of human history, and for the majority of human beings, that default setting - a.k.a. "ye ol' in 'n' out" - was about all there was. And, it worked. Sort of. Women may not have had a lot of orgasms from that. But, most women didn't even know such things existed. They still got a nice chemical cocktail. It just wasn't the level of an orgasm.

Then we got vibrators.

Wait, let me back up. First we added a bunch of other stuff. We have phallic shaped devices going back to ancient times discovered in archeological digs all over the world in almost every culture. Cleopatra is even rumoured to have had a device that would be filled with bees for a little vibration. And then we started getting creative about what we were doing to each others genitals. Oral sex, digital manipulation, erotica... There's no cave art for any of that, but we can be sure it has been a long history of creativity.

I would love to know when the first blowjob occurred. When did that happen and how did that go the first time some man brought that up?

"You want to put it WHERE?"

"In your mouth."

"With all my teeth?"

"Yeah. No. Don't actually 'eat' it. Just like 'down there' but, you know, with your mouth."

(shrugs) "Okay. But wash it first."

I read a story about a woman who felt so empowered when she bought her first vibrator. She used a fake ID at an adult store when she was still a teenager. She was still learning about how to have an orgasm, through any means. But once she got the vibrator and put it to her clit, angels sang. Suddenly, she was able to have a dozen orgasms back to back any time she wanted. Life was great.

And when a man entered the picture, she made sure he was okay with her using her vibrator on her clit while they had sex. He was. Life was great.

Then it wasn't. Just like the woman who spent her tax refunds, eventually, the vibrators didn't work anymore.

The first problem was that she got bored with the vibrator. It was the ONLY way she could get off and even new types of vibrators were still the same ol' thing. And then they stopped working so automatically. Even with her favorite vibrator, it was taking her longer and longer to reach orgasm. And then it got to where she could hardly orgasm at all. Without an orgasm, she lost interest in sex altogether. It was depressing. And, you can imagine the work she had to do to straighten that out.

For men, do just about anything with the penis and it triggers an orgasm response. For women, it was probably like that at one point in human history. Do just about anything with her genitals and BAM!! Thousands of years of slut-shaming and repression have made that much more complicated nowadays. But, the cause and effect is still technically the same, even when it doesn't work.

For women who have become dependent on their vibrator for orgasms, their orgasm response is actually more like men. It has become like a necessary chore to "get done" and then be done with it. That's often how men masturbate. Where's the playing and all the time spent on the journey? Gone. Why waste time with all that? Gimme my orgasm and give it to me now. Life is great.

Until it isn't.

Technically speaking, until you start robbing liquor stores for money to buy vibrators, or turning tricks on the street corner, or stealing from your family and friends, or pawning your shit for pennies on the dollar, it really doesn't reach the bar to be classified as an addiction.

It's a dependency. That's different. A dependency is when you are "dependent" on the vibrator to achieve the desired effect. You can be addicted to masturbating. Dependency is when all that masturbating doesn't do you any good without a vibrator. This may sound like semantics, but it is really is different.

For many women, their first orgasm was a happy accident. Many had their first orgasm while touching themselves. And for a while, there was some learning to make that happen NOT by accident. And going forward, the vibrator got added later, after some time spent just playing with yourself and figuring things out. If you are unable to masturbate and orgasm with just your fingers and some alone time, you have possibly become dependent.

If you can only orgasm with a vibrator, you are limiting your sexual experience. Virtually every part of a woman's body is capable of bringing her to orgasm. There are THOUSANDS of different types of orgasms and THOUSANDS of different ways to experience pleasure. Why would you funnel it down to one very procedural activity and stop exploring all those other possibilities?

I heard it described like sexual fast food. It's kinda delicious and efficient for filling the belly. But, we all know it isn't healthy and it isn't deeply satisfying. Vibrators are like that. The orgasms are wonderful and satisfying. But also not healthy (overall) and deeply satisfying. There's nothing wrong with a Whopper sometimes, or some Chicken McNuggets. But not every meal. The same thing applies to using a vibrator.

So many teenagers are shamed against masturbating. Women especially. Being able to "rub one out" often leaves a girl with embarrassment and shame. So, the quicker you can get it done, the better. Fingers simply don't accomplish the goal as quickly and efficiently. A vibrator is so efficient that it temporarily removes the guilt and shame. It doesn't work nearly as well as developing healthy attitudes about sex, but it works. In a way, a vibrator eliminates the need to work on healthy sexuality. Masturbating with the exploratory method can trigger all those feelings. Who has time for that?

Vibrators work so well that you don't have to be "in the mood", physically or mentally. You can be watching TV or thinking about work or your kids and the vibrator will still make it happen quickly and efficiently. There's a comfort zone to it.

This works and gets the job done and you can continue to feel capable and that everything is fine. Until… It stops working.

Not every woman becomes dependent. Even some that use a vibrator every day or every time they have sex. But truthfully, it's impossible to place a number on the ones that do. I mean, how many women are taking surveys on this? How many women are talking to their doctor or therapist about this? How many are actually seeking help for this, once they figure out that it's a problem? Right. So, I'm guessing the percentage of women who become dependent is somewhere between none and all of them. (grins and shrugs)

You're the only one who can decide. Think about your life WITHOUT a vibrator. What would that look like? If it looks like the end of your sex life, you have possibly become dependent. You're also the only one who can decide if this is a problem you want to correct. Some women are quite happy and don't want to change it. It's up to you.

The thing is, women experience sex cognitively. Satisfying the body and triggering the orgasm response in the brain as quickly as possible might feel great. But, it completely bypasses the natural way a woman experiences orgasm. If you remove what is natural, how long do you think it will take for the body to rebel? And that is what happens. Eventually, even the body cannot make it happen with the greatest tool we have ever developed for that purpose.

If you have become dependent, you are not lost. There is hope. And the treatment is A LOT of fun. Well, at first, it will be insanely frustrating. But then, it will be fun. Don't throw your vibrators out. Keep them. Vibrators are awesome!! Just… Put them away for a while.

How do you fix it? See the REBOOT article in this series, coming up next.

Part 8:
REBOOT!!

So. Why don't you cum?

Stop masturbating like men. (drops mic)

(picks mic back up)

A party for one is still a party, and you need to learn how to party right. Studies show that less than 10% of women masturbate regularly. For whatever reason - and there are many - they aren't doing the ONE thing that will help them have a better sex life in every way. And not just a better sex life, but a better life overall.

* Orgasms release a wonderful chemical cocktail into the system. As stated earlier, the cocktail consists of oxytocin, serotonin, dopamine, melatonin, vasopressin, some nitric oxide and some prolactin, plus small doses of a few others that are healthy for you. This cocktail makes you happy and gives you peace. And, there is a growing body of evidence that it cures damn near everything else.

* Women who masturbate regularly are more comfortable with their bodies in a healthy way. When you have some self acceptance with your body, an amazing thing happens: you are more likely to take care of yourself in other ways.

* Self acceptance leads to self confidence. Imagine how your WHOLE LIFE will improve with an improved level of self confidence. Will it effect your career? Yes. Will it effect your relationships? Yes. Will it bring you millions? Probably not. But, you'll have the confidence to do the

work that will make you more successful in every area of your life.

*   Masturbating will empower your sex life. You will have a better understanding of your body and what she needs. Your confidence will help you express to your lover what you need. You'll be able to communicate better in intimate ways. And, it will help you make better decisions in your relationships, which means lovers who work WITH you, not against you.

*   Even if you are not in a relationship, masturbating will keep your sexuality healthy for when you do include a partner. Think of it like practicing for the game. Between the body and the brain, masturbating will maintain great sexual response.

*   Are you tired? Stressed? Depressed? The chemicals released when you masturbate regularly will help regulate your sleep much, much better and completely relieve stress. It greatly improves depression. You'll also see your digestive system get better. Your immune system will improve. It will even help your skin clear up a little. I read a small, independent study that showed women's hair got healthier when they masturbate regularly.

    Some scientists have even found evidence that it improves cognition and may reduce the likelihood of Alzheimer's. There's a lot of evidence that it helps prevent cancer throughout the entire body. Every kind of cancer.

*   Especially in women, masturbating can ease chronic pain. From headaches, to back aches, all types of pain are eased with the chemical cocktail. All the heavy breathing might even help clear up your sinuses.

*   Masturbating, especially from internal stimulation, can relieve menstrual cramps. Almost instantaneously, and they might be gone for the rest of your cycle.

Yes, I'm being a bit light hearted with all this. But the truth is, we don't even know ALL the ways oxytocin and the rest of cocktail improves health. We just know that it does in virtually every way.

And best of all, there are no side effects. There has yet to be a single discovery of ANY negatives to oxytocin and the rest of the sex chemicals. Not one.

And since you are capable of having as many orgasms as you want, any time you want, why are you not doing that? There should be mandated masturbation breaks at work to improve morale and productivity. Can't cum? Bullshit!!

So. Masturbate passionately and often. Just don't do it like men. Goal oriented and "chore-like". Do it like a Goddess!!

Start by going back to basics. Remember the first time you touched yourself? Start there. I suggest a masturbation exercise that has two parts. How you masturbate teaches your body what to recognize as pleasure. So, let's teach your body that there is an I-N-F-I-N-I-T-E range to the pleasure it is capable of experiencing and teach your body to break free from limitations.

Part one will make it sound like I am canceling everything I just said in some of the other parts of this series. LOL!!

REBOOT
for a single woman

First thing in the morning, masturbate and give yourself an orgasm. Do it as quickly as possible. Get it done. Use whatever you have to use, even a vibrator. Get it done.

Don't have time? Bullshit! Make time. Get it done.

You have other things going on in the morning? Getting kids off to school. Getting yourself off to work? Make time to get yourself off. This is not supposed to be a long, drawn out thing. Get it done as quickly as possible. Make the time and get it done.

If you try and can't get yourself there, that's okay. When you reach the point where you know it isn't going to happen, move on with your day and don't worry about it. Try again the next day. Yes, I know you'll likely be frustrated and cranky. That's okay too. I promise, this will get better if you keep trying.

One benefit aside from the reboot is that you'll go to work with your system full of oxytocin, which just makes you more peaceful and relaxed all day. That isn't part of the exercise and not part of the goal. It's just a nice extra.

Part two is when the magic happens. We're going to bookend your sexual responses with the other ends of a very wide spectrum. This time, there is no goal to "get it done". You are not trying to have an orgasm. There is no time limit. There is no goal except to explore.

Turn off everything. No TV. No computer. No phone. No porn. No vibrator!! I even suggest turning off the lights to avoid visual stimulation. This part is just you and your brain. And your fingers.

Turn the brain off. I know. Harder than it sounds. It might take practice.

If you want to take a warm bath first to relax, that's not a bad idea. A glass of wine is also not a bad idea. Not too much. Being intoxicated will be counter productive. Get naked, relax in bed and get physically comfortable.

Start by feeling the sheets against your skin. Feel the way your body lays there. Feel the liberation of your own nakedness.

Then start slowly, gently touching yourself. Start with your face and hair and neck. Feel your touch and feel how it feels to be touched so lovingly. This exercise is for exploration and self love. It is for re-discovery and re-connection to your sexual self in a loving, nurturing, KIND way.

S-L-O-W-L-Y work your way down to your breasts. The breasts have so many possibilities for pleasure. Don't hurry. Touch the sides. Touch the bottom of your breasts. Touch between them. It's easy to go for the nipples right away. But, be patient. Explore the infinite possibilities around them. This exercise is the truest essence of self love. Be patient. There is no goal. There is no hurry to get to that goal.

Something that might help is to create a mantra you can recite to yourself as you're doing this to help focus the brain and eliminate distracting thoughts. "Love," for example. "I'm doing this to show myself some love," is an example. You can even tell yourself, "I love you" because with this exercise, you are showing yourself that you do.

Touch your stomach and sides. Don't love your body? Understandable. Many people don't. But this is your body, as is. Love her. Touch her.

Skip the juicy bits for now and go down to your legs, and even your feet. Touch them. Love them. Gentle and nurturing. Fat thighs? Fine. Love them anyway. They are part of you, as is. To love YOU is to accept YOU. This exercise is for self acceptance.

When you get to the good stuff, it is common for women to focus on her clitoris and nothing else. You actually have a phazillion other pleasure places. Why limit yourself? For this exercise, you must explore more than the clitoris. Feel. Everything. Feel the entire vulva. Feel the labia, inner and outer. Feel the vaginal opening, the vestibule. Feel the intense pleasure of first entering your vagina with your fingers. Feel it all. Play with your labia like you love it. Find you g-spot. Feel for your cervix. Feel everything.

As I said, the goal here is not to have an orgasm. If it happens, fine. Wonderful. But that is actually not the goal. The goal is simply to feel and explore and learn the very light touch of your fingers. Make your nerve endings work with softness. Teach them to feel everything. Every subtle detail.

And, feel it emotionally. Let go of thought and just let yourself feel. No hurry. No end game. Do this as long as it takes. You'll know when you are done for the night.

What this does is create a bookend of sexual pleasure response. You will get in touch with your body and your soul. You will train your brain that ALL of it is pleasure and you will be able to experience pleasure from a full range of stimulation.

This type of masturbation - the type you engaged in at first contact - will give you self acceptance, which will give you self confidence. As we know, confidence brings joys and benefits aplenty.

REBOOT
for a woman in a sexual relationship

This is a little more complicated for women who are in a relationship, but not too much. The two steps above are still the core of this REBOOT. You will still do those. Part two off the exercise above will be a challenge with someone sharing your bed to sleep. But, work it out. There's always a way if you're willing.

In addition to those two exercises, start with communication with your partner. Have a deep, honest conversation about what you're doing. If your partner isn't on board, that's something to think about. Tell your partner that you're doing this to revive your sexual pleasure, but also your sexuality and yourSELF. Let your partner know this isn't about them. It is for you.

And second, when you have sex with that partner, no vibrators for a while. Learn to use your own mind to connect sexually. Learn to use your fingers and hands to rebuild the pleasure response naturally. Encourage your partner to use their fingers and hands to explore your body like never before. Feel everything. Every sensation. Every touch. Every subtle detail.

S-L-O-W D-O-W-N!! Encourage your partner to explore with you. Slow everything down and focus on sensations. This exercise can seem very selfish to your partner and feel (to them) that you are excluding them from something important in your life. So, include them. Not at first. You need to practice a little before you do that. But soon.

Loooooooooong drawn out simmering and foreplay sessions are important. Just touch and use your mind to connect to your body. Feel. Everything. And show your partner how.

When you reach a point where you can regularly orgasm from touch by itself, you can break out the vibrators again. But, not every time. Expand what you do in bed and each time, incorporate your fingers and hands and touch. I'll say it again, feel everything. Explore the full range of female sexual pleasure and you'll enjoy rewards that will make your sex life incredible.

The REBOOT exercise might take a month, it might take the rest of your life. However, women who masturbate in a loving way, without a goal, are infinitely happier and healthier in ALL areas of their lives, in bed and out.

Women who can masturbate without the goal are seldom wondering why they can't cum. Jus' sayin'.